Asthma.

If I can recover, you can too.

A physician shares his own journey.

ISBN: 978-1-62209-515-5

ISBN-13: 978-1481187046

ISBN-10: 148118704X

Cover graphics graciously provided by

Genova Diagnostics.

Contents

Chapter 1
If I can recover, you can too

Hello, my name is Robert Murdoch. I am a physician practicing all holistic medicine in Southwest Florida, and consulting with patients from all over the world.

I used to have asthma. By using specific, deliberate steps, I overcame it. I did it, many of my patients have done it, and you can do it too.

Here's my story: I was born and raised in Sherwood Forest. Yes, there is such a place. No, I didn't know Robin Hood, I'm not THAT old! I grew up with two older brothers and three younger sisters. Most of my childhood we lived in the countryside outside of a small village called Wellow, in a house surrounded by fields and woodlands. It was a beautiful setting in the summer. A little bleak in the winter. My Mother, Marie-Antoinette would say how cold it was in that house in the winter. I don't remember. I remember making mud pies with my sister on the driveway, and making dens in the woods, chasing rats in the barns, walking miles with our dog, Buck.

My father, Denis, was an architect. He worked in Nottingham. He had asthma, eczema and intermittent bronchitis. I guess I copied some of his traits.

When I was a child, I was sick most of the time; I felt weak. I felt cold right through my belly. Often I couldn't breathe. I missed half my primary schooling through sickness. I'd been diagnosed with asthma, severe hay fever allergies, eczema and chronic bronchitis.

Here's how it felt when things were bad: take a 5mm diameter straw, and breathe through it... for 2 days. Exhausting? Yes! Debilitating? You bet! Because you're reading this, you probably already know what that's like, or you know someone who does. The greatest relief I got was sleep. I didn't ever know if I was going to die in my sleep, but I was willing to give up the hard work needed to breathe and to stay alive, just to get some rest, not knowing if I was going to wake up, and really being too tired to care. The prescription bronchiodilator sprays would help, but I needed to take them 2 - 7 times per day, everyday for about 16 years.

I also had eczema. I remember looking at the inside of elbows, and backs of knees of my schoolmates and thinking "So that's how normal skin looks!" I can vividly remember my mother saying "Don't scratch!" I would do my best not to scratch, but it felt so good when I did, then it would bleed, and hurt more. A little more scratching relieved it, then more bleeding, and more pain. We would use the corticosteroid creams, which made my skin paper-thin and made the pores disappear for several years.

Over the years, I had round after round of antibiotics. They sometimes helped in the short term.

Around the age of eighteen, I discovered natural medicine. I tried the Bach Flower Remedies, hands on healing, homeopathy, diet changes, and then... acupuncture. I met Brian Thomas, a Welshman, who was graduating from The College of Traditional Chinese Acupuncture. He introduced me to the whole notion that the "Terrain is decisive". In other words, diseases can't exist in a strong, healthy person. First of all it was Brian Thomas treated me with acupuncture, then Susan Woodhead, then John Hicks. Acupuncture really changed my life. Instead of merely stopping symptoms, it actually helped build my health; a concept quite foreign to me until that point. My hay fever allergies disappeared, I developed healthy lungs, and my skin healed completely. This fascinating system of medicine helped my health so much that I also took it on as a career.

While I was in the process of having my courses of acupuncture treatment, I noticed that a certain Homeopathic remedy also helped my breathing, along with dietary changes and nutritional supplementation. I found the value of eliminating allergenic foods from my diet, and of eating whole foods. These methods would reduce, and for the most part, eliminate relapses.

I remember my first encounter with higher doses of vitamin C. I had been on three consecutive courses of antibiotics for bronchitis/pneumonia over a period of a month. There had been no improvement. Someone suggested five grams of vitamin C per day. I took it and in two days I was completely better.

Years later, I met the legendary Archivides (Archie) Kalokerinos MD, a very funny and profoundly compassionate man, who had saved thousands of lives by the administration of Vitamin C. I encourage you to look him up.

Then there were vaccines; yes, after getting myself healthy by the age of 25, I took polio and tetanus boosters. Guess what…sick again, just in the same way I was when I was as a child. I found myself thinking "All those years of sickness were from vaccines? Damn!"

Having learned how to recover and detoxify, I was able to do that once more, but this time much more quickly. That started me on my long and in-depth journey of investigating vaccines.

Then there were mercury/silver dental amalgam fillings. You know, I really wonder what happened when that first someone thought "Ah! Tooth decay, let's drill it out and, okay... let's fill the hole with something containing... let me think... let's see... how about...MERCURY! Yes mercury should do the trick!"? Somehow that **"No! STOP! THAT'S A REALLY BAD IDEA!"** filter that most of us have in our brains, just didn't kick in. Nope, those thoughts to put mercury in teeth were actually implemented. And it has taken this many years and hoards of people with at least an ounce of knowledge about science to point out that **THIS IS A PROBLEM!** Later in this book, I will discuss the relationship between heavy metal toxicity and asthma.

As for me, I eventually had all my mercury fillings removed, and had some chelation therapy, which we'll also discuss later.

When I was 22 years old, my 21-year-old sister, Anita, whom we all called "Popette", was traveling through France with a friend. They stopped at a restaurant. Part way through the meal Popette started experiencing an asthma attack. In the process of straining to breathe, she vomited. She aspirated the vomit, choked and died. While Popette's death was an indirect result of asthma, I hope it serves all of us as a reminder to be diligent in building good health, and of course being well trained and ready with first aid procedures.

As for me, I regained my health. I know that if I can do it from where I was, you can too. And you can help your loved ones do the same. In this book I'll share each component of it.

I want you and yours to be healthy. I want you to live a full life, to fulfill your objectives, to live the life you were born to live. To that end I became a physician, practicing acupuncture, Oriental medicine, homeopathy, functional medicine, nutritional counseling, and NLP.

During my decades of being in practice, I spent four years in Dallas. In that time I had the distinct privilege to work with Dr. Michael Samuels. Dr. Samuels is a Doctor of Osteopathy with a genius intellect. He practiced medicine in a way I'd never seen until that point. He included homeopathy, nutritional counseling, chelation therapy, cranio-sacral therapy, and modern, allopathic medicine.

What characterized his practice was shrewd insight, compassion, pragmatism, and a relentless drive to find underlying causes.

Dr. Samuels didn't know it at the time, but he influenced my approach to medicine in such a way that what I have learned, both from him and from my studies inspired by his approach, has helped thousands of people.

In my practice, just like every medical/health practitioner around the world, I have favorite patients and favorite conditions with which I like to work. With my own health history, one of my favorite conditions to help a patient to resolve, is asthma. To qualify that remark, I have to say that having the label "Asthma" as a diagnosis, is of no use in recovery, because it has so many different causes. Recognizing the cause is useful as long as there is a successful resolution.

In this book I've included a variety of approaches and tools that you can use to become healthy. (Please don't tell me "I am healthy apart from this asthma." Healthy people don't have asthma. Really. Healthy people don't have diseases, period.)

Whatever herbs, nutritionals, drugs, or homeopathics you have been using to keep your condition tolerable, stay on them for now. As your health improves, work with your prescribing doctor(s) to adjust dosages appropriate to your new state of health.

Chapter 2
What is asthma?

❖ It is the spasming of the smaller tubes that carry air into the lungs (bronchioles). This reduces the amount of air that can pass through the tubes and into and out of the lungs.

❖ It is the inflammation and consequent swelling of the mucus membranes in the lungs. Once again, this swelling reduces the amount of air that can pass in and out of the lungs.

And a few extra facts:

❖ Often but not always, extra mucus is produced, and sometimes there is enough extra mucus to further block the airways.

❖ Asthma is often mild, and without treatment, prevents a person from reaching their full athletic potential. At the other end of the spectrum, asthma can be lethal. The bronchioles (small tubes in the lungs) can close up to the extent that insufficient oxygen is absorbed by the body to stay alive. Most asthmatics have mild asthma, but many do have moderate intensity asthma, and of course many have severe episodes.

❖ During episodes, asthmatics generally reduce their activity, focus on forcefully taking deeper breaths, pulling air in and pushing air out, often bracing their arms on a nearby object - a wall, a counter top, or on their thighs, so that the pectoralis major chest muscles help the movement of the ribs.

❖ There are a variety of triggers for an episode, for instance: viral, bacterial or fungal infection, inhaled dust, smoke or pollen, solvents, perfumes, cleaning products, nervousness, anxiety or emotional upset, exercise, allergic reaction to food, to drugs or to other airborne allergens.

According to the CDC:
   ❖ In 2009, one in 12 people had asthma, that's 12 million people in the US.
   ❖ In 2007 asthma cost around $56 billion per year, in the US alone.
   ❖ 185 children and 3,262 adults died from asthma in 2007.

Chapter 3
What Causes Asthma?

Mental & emotional components

Please, please, please don't underestimate the roll of emotions in health. I know that modern, allopathic medicine likes to compartmentalize parts of the human being through what is referred to as 'specialization', and of course psychology and psychiatry are areas that study and treat the mind, the emotions and the brain. In my opinion, the vast majority of interactions back and forth between the whole body and mind, are ignored by modern allopathic medicine. In other words, there are far more thoughts and mental states that express themselves as physical symptoms than most physicians recognize. Conversely, there are far more mental and emotional states that are caused by dietary, drug and environmental influences than most physicians recognize. It's a huge and dreadful oversight.

Let's look at a few of the emotions that can cause problems:

❖ Fear
❖ Anger/frustration
❖ Shock

- ❖ Heartbreak
- ❖ Over excitement
- ❖ Worry
- ❖ Grief

Any of these can be enough to have a person become asthmatic, if they hold the tension from the emotion in their chest. They can be a contributory factor of either the initial onset of asthma, or of an asthmatic episode. The tension produced in the body in these situations can manifest in the muscles surrounding the airways, reducing airflow, and in the muscles around the chest and diaphragm.

I remember many times when I was asthmatic, when I'd go out feeling fine, until I realized that I'd left my inhaler at home. Right away, my lungs would tighten up. It sounds crazy to people who haven't experienced it. I can imagine them thinking "Just don't think that way." But it takes training and practice.

I remember one of my patients in Dallas was admitted to hospital, into the pulmonary department. She had difficulty breathing. I went to visit. I asked about the onset of the episode. After a few questions, she revealed that she and her husband had had an argument minutes before the onset. This is surprisingly common.

Fungus and antibiotics

There are very few physicians who even consider that fungal infections can exist in the lungs, but I assert that most, but not all, asthma is at least in part a result of fungal infections in the lungs. And my opinion is borne out by clinical observations in many patients.

Fungus can be inhaled into the lungs, or travel from the intestines, through the blood stream to the lungs.

A pattern that occurs for so many people is this: they get a bacterial infection, they get antibiotics, the antibiotics kill the harmful bacteria, the antibiotics also kill the good bacteria. Now, it is still warm and wet in the intestines, lungs, sinuses, sex organs, skin. Something is going to grow. Women know that vaginal fungal/yeast/thrush infections often occur after antibiotics. But remember, fungi are not perverts, they will live anywhere that is warm and wet. Add sugar, and fungus grows double fast. The lungs are also warm and wet, so fungus is just as likely to grow in there.

Fungal infections can stay in an individual for decades.

When fungus gets into the lungs it irritates the mucus membranes, makes them swell, increases their mucus production, and makes them very sensitive indeed to particles (dust, pollen, smoke, etc.).

How do you know if you have fungus in your lungs? You can test for fungus a few ways. Methods 2, 3 and 4 are not specific to your lungs:

1. **Sputum analysis.** This is the best way to test.
2. **Stool analysis**. This can be accurate for types and levels of fungus in the body, but if we use it as a diagnosis for lung fungus we'd be making an educated guess.
3. **Blood antibodies.** Not so accurate. It doesn't tell you the current status of fungus in the body.
4. **Live blood cell analysis by microscopy.** This has a similar level of accuracy as the stool analysis, except that we can't determine which type of fungus we're looking at, and we can't do sensitivity tests (these are tests that check which antifungal/antimicrobial tests will work well).

Environmental challenges

- ❖ *Mold/fungus.* This is worse in certain parts of the world. More humid and damp places provide better breeding ground for fungus. There are, of course buildings that have more fungus/mold than others.
- ❖ *Dust mites.* These feed on house dust, most of which is flakes of human skin. Dust mites eat the skin, then they poop, and their poop is a common allergen that causes respiratory difficulty.
- ❖ *Dust.* There are many minute particles that float in the air at home, at places of work, and at construction and demolition sites.
- ❖ *Pollen.* Especially at certain times of the year, pollen is released by plants to "impregnate" other plants of the same species. The pollen from certain plants floats in the air, and we breathe it in.
- ❖ *Solvents and cleaning chemicals.* Whether at home or at work, these can be tough on the lungs.
- ❖ *Pollution, smoke and soot.* Second hand smoke, vehicle exhaust fumes, industrial exhaust, fires, and smoke and dust from volcanic eruptions. These do vary substantially from place to place. In some areas, breathing the air is quite unsafe.

Any of these can, when they come into contact with the mucus membranes of the lungs, cause irritation, and then inflammation. This irritation can cause the mucus membranes to produce more mucus, which can reduce airflow to the lungs, and to have the small muscles around the bronchioles contract.

Dietary habits

Allergies and food sensitivities:

There are certain foods that can cause or contribute to asthma. There are foods that are considered allergens, and some that, in certain individuals, cause a negative reaction that is not technically an allergy. You might call these situations "intolerances" or "sensitivities". An allergy is a situation where the immune system inappropriately produces antibodies against something that, for most people, is innocuous.

The food allergen that affects more people than any other is gluten. Gluten is a protein in certain grains. It is most plentiful in wheat. It also occurs in rye, barley, and more obscure grains: spelt, kamut, amaranth, and triticale. It is also found as a result of cross-contamination in other foods processed in the same food factories and mills.

Gluten does not usually cause a problem for the lungs. But in a few people it does, and for some it is a big problem.

My daughter suffered lungfuls of bubbly phlegm that would be triggered only by gluten, and would only be cleared up by the removal of gluten from her diet, AND with the administration of a particular homeopathic. But if she'd have gluten again, she'd have more phlegm.

The food group that creates more problems for asthmatics than any other, is dairy. Mention problems with dairy and most people think of lactose intolerance, and heart disease from dairy fats. Lactose rarely, if ever causes any respiratory problems. Dairy fats rarely, if ever causes any respiratory problems.

Why dairy really and powerfully impacts respiratory function is that the proteins in dairy irritate the mucus membranes of the body, including the mucus membranes of the lungs. The lining of the lungs inflame, and they produce more mucus. Dairy proteins are known to create an autoimmune response.

According to the Food Allergy and Anaphylaxis Network, 90% of all food allergies are to the following foods

1. Milk
2. Egg
3. Peanut
4. Tree nuts
5. Fish
6. Shellfish
7. Soy
8. Wheat

I agree with them, but I would expand the description as follows:

1. Dairy in general, including as ingredients to other foods. Dairy is VERY OFTEN a cause of asthma, or worsens it.
2. Egg. Eggs rarely, but sometimes are a problem for asthmatics.
3. Peanuts (actually a legume) can restrict breathing through anaphylaxis.
4. Tree nuts. Occasionally a problem for asthmatics.
5. Fish. Occasionally a problem for asthmatics.
6. Shellfish. Occasionally a problem for asthmatics.
7. Soy. Rarely a problem for asthmatics.
8. All gluten grains and derivatives thereof. Gluten is sometimes a problem for asthmatics.

It's also important to remember that most food processing facilities allow cross-contamination from one food product to another, either through surfaces and containers that are inadequately cleaned, or through dust in the processing plant.

To claim a product is gluten-free, it needs to have been tested at 20 or fewer parts per million (ppm). There are many products that are sold as gluten free, which are above that, up as high as 500ppm. To make a comparison: regular bread is 10,000ppm.

Take the initiative, call food manufacturers, ask them to see the written results of the ELISA testing they've had performed. If they don't have this information for you, they are only guessing at the levels of any of the allergens in their products.

Non-Organic foods:

When you consider that agricultural topsoil is depleted by approximately 85% of most nutrient minerals, in comparison to how it was in 1930 (Organic farms, of course maintain much fuller nutrient density in their soils.) It's easy to see why foods in grocery stores just do not have enough minerals, vitamins or proteins to sustain a healthy body. Like every system in the body, the lungs, the nerves and immune system all need good nutrition to function well.

Another factor to remember about conventionally (non-organically) grown food is that it contains chemical fertilizers, herbicides, pesticides and fungicides, all of which put extra toxic burden on the body. They irritate and deteriorate organs and tissues and they need to be gotten out of the body, and kept out. In order for the liver to remove these toxins, it requires more of the essential nutrients that are absent in the foods carrying the toxins. Through this, conventionally grown foods are a double threat!

Refined foods:

Refined foods deplete the body of nutrients. Many amino acids, vitamins and minerals are needed to digest and process foods in the body. Whole, organically grown foods give back to the body more than they take out, providing raw materials for all the body's functions, repair and fuel. Refined foods don't do that, they take without giving back.

And sugar. What is yeast/fungus's favorite food? Sugar! If you're eating a diet high in sugar, even high in fruit, you will be feeding fungus. If that fungus happens to be in the lungs: trouble!

<u>Infections</u>

We all know that besides fungus, there are viruses and bacteria that love to find a home in the lungs. Some are harmless, some are a nuisance, some are dangerous, and some are deadly. The harmful ones produce toxins that are a challenge to the body's detoxification system. Of course the physiological response you have to those microbes depends upon the strength of your immune system, the level of your nutrition, and a few other factors.

Once you deal with the acute infection, and gain stability you may fully recover. On the other hand there may be some residual lung inflammation. Often corticosteroids are prescribed to clear the inflammation, but sometimes there is a residual spasm, with phlegm and inflammation in the lungs that continues.

<u>Vaccines</u>

I have several concerns about vaccines:

1. Vaccines contain mercury, aluminum, formaldehyde, and organic, inorganic, live and dead contaminants. In fact, some of the microbes in the vaccines are not meant to be in there, like for instance the SV 40 and the SIV in the polio vaccines that ended up causing cancer (SV40), and HIV (mutated from the SIV) in millions of people. While the vaccine believers will say that it's okay to have these toxins in vaccines, and that it's okay to inject them into babies and small children, and that most children who are vaccinated survive and are seemingly unhurt, I assert that it's impossible to inject those substances without at least some detrimental effect.

2. 1 in every 68 children in US schools in 2010 had a diagnosis within the autism spectrum disorder (ASD). Whereas unvaccinated children are diagnosed at a rate of less than 1 in 1000 ASD. We are told "The link between vaccines and autism has been disproved", I am curious…disproved by who? When? Which studies have disproved it? Once again, they don't come forward with statistics, or independent studies.

3. Autism is far from the only danger of vaccines: allergies, asthma (more than double the rate of unvaccinated children), dementia, hyperactivity, seizures, and death (often diagnosed as SIDS, and the so-called "shaken baby syndrome").

4. The diseases for which vaccines were developed had declined by 70-90+% from the 1800's prior to the introduction of the vaccines (See the US Department of the Census vital statistics, and the British Commonwealth Yearbook, and the Vital Statistics of England and Wales).

5. There are outbreaks in vaccinated populations. Vaccinated individuals don't do any better in an outbreak than unvaccinated. The largest clinical trial ever done on any medicine proves this. The University of Michigan, 1955, Francis, et al's study on the Salk polio vaccine. It was done on over 1,000,000 children, with 750,000 children used as placebo. During the 6 months of the study, an average of 57 of every 100,000 vaccinated children got polio, and 54 of every 100,000 children in the placebo group got polio. You might say "Well, polio disappeared after the vaccine was released, so it must have worked." In actual fact, polio was reclassified in 1957. The diagnostic criteria were changed to exclude over 95% of cases. People

who fell within the earlier diagnostic parameters were no longer to be diagnosed with polio, they had 'Aseptic meningitis' which later became called 'Viral meningitis'. So at that point, polio rates plummeted, and aseptic meningitis rates went through the roof.

6. According to the US CDC, FDA, the World Health Organization and so many other so called "Health" organizations, the measure of vaccine effectiveness is not immunity, but antibodies produced after administration. I know, I know, we have a cultural belief that antibodies equal immunity. But if they really did, everyone with HIV, hepatitis, herpes, brucellosis, malaria, dange, Epstein-Barr virus (another herpes), all these people and others would be cured, because they have the antibodies, they'd be immune. But they are all susceptible to the disease. Antibodies do not equal immunity. And in fact, it is this very elevation in antibodies caused by the antigens and the aluminum in the vaccines that are among the most powerful contributors to allergic reactions, including asthma.

One problem with believing what the people at the FDA, CDC, WHO, etc. say, and following their recommendations, is that every single employee at each of those organizations is allowed to own stock in drug companies. They are allowed to have jobs with drug companies. Then of course, there is the revolving door. Do a favor for a drug company, and you might just get a really good job with them. It's a degree of corruption you might expect to see in a third world country, but we have it here and now, and our children are taking the brunt of it.

And no, you don't have to be vaccinated to get into school, employment, or the military. They will usually lie to make you think you do, but there are legal exemptions available to you. Find out which exemptions are available in your area.

Metal toxicity

This is not usually considered an issue by most physicians, but if they knew how and why this causes problems they'd be straight onto it. Not only are metals such as mercury (Hg), aluminium (aluminum) (Al), and lead (Pb) neurotoxins, and need to be expelled from the body, they make the body very susceptible to infection. They do this by breaking up heme. Heme is a part of hemoglobin. When heme is broken up, it allows free iron to circulate, and fungus and bacteria LOVE free iron. If you have lung problems, it is a nightmare to be susceptible to infection, but unfortunately, it is very common.

Where do we get metal toxicity? Many heavy metals can be passed on to us from our mothers. So for instance, if your mother has mercury dental amalgams, she could have unwittingly passed metal toxicity to you while she was pregnant with you.

Common sources:

Deodorant:	Aluminium (Aluminum)
Drink cans:	Aluminium (Aluminum)
Baking powder:	Aluminium (Aluminum)
Salt:	Aluminium (Aluminum)
Vaccines:	Mercury and Aluminium (Aluminum)
Amalgam fillings:	Mercury

Shellfish: Arsenic

Fish & fish oils: Mercury

Tobacco & marijuana: Cadmium

Aluminum cookware: Aluminium (Aluminum)

Certain food colorings: Aluminium (Aluminum). Aluminium food color exists in some thyroid medications, which is so ironic, because aluminium blocks the body's thyroxin receptors.

How do you know if you have these metals in your body? There are several lab tests that detect toxic metals in the body, these include:

1. Hair analysis -

   Pros: Easy to collect

   Cons: Depends a lot on the body's ability to detoxify itself, the better it detoxifies, and the less the metals bind to the body's tissues, the more metal is likely to show up in the hair, and vice versa.

2. Blood analysis

   Pros:

   Cons: If the metals are bound to the body's tissues, they won't show up in the blood.

3. Challenged or provoked blood analysis

Pros: Metals will show according to which agent (or substance) is used to challenge/ provoke/ chelate, (i.e. to pull it out of storage, into circulation), the dosage of the agent, and the time between the dosage and collecting the sample. All these factors need to be consistent from one sample to another, especially in the same patient.

Cons: We have to keep the chelating agent, its dosage and the time between dosage and collection consistent. Different chelating agents are efficient for different metals, so which to use for the test is an issue. Also, it takes drawing blood, a problem with some patients.

4. Urine analysis

Pros: Easy to collect.

Cons: If the metals are bound to the body's tissues, they won't show up in the urine, and mercury rarely shows in the urine.

5. Challenged or provoked urine analysis

Pros: Easy to collect. Just like in the blood, metals will show up according to which agent (or substance) is used to challenge/provoke/chelate, (i.e. to pull it out of storage, into circulation), the dosage of the agent, and the time between the dosage and collecting the sample. All these factors need to be consistent from one sample to another, especially in the same patient.

Cons: We have to keep the chelating agent, its dosage and the time between dosage and collection consistent. Different chelating agents are efficient for different metals, so which to use for the test is an issue, and most mercury is excreted through the stool.

6. Stool analysis:

   Pros: Easy, and delightful to collect. Mercury is much more likely to show up in the stool than in urine.

   Cons: If the metals are bound to the body's tissues rather than circulating, they won't show up in the stool.

7. Urinary porphyrins. This is the method I use, as recommended by the world's leading authority on heavy metal toxicity in humans, Professor Boyd Haley.

   Pros: Easy to collect. Challenge/ provocation/ chelation prior to test is not required.

   Cons: Only shows the presence of arsenic, lead, aluminum and mercury (but these are the most important ones to know about in the prevention of bacterial and fungal overgrowths in your body).

TREATMENTS SECTION

Chapter 4

Modern, allopathic treatments

Health agencies and modern allopaths will tell you that there is no cure for asthma. Why would they say that? To find out, I recommend you follow the money. While most of those individuals are well-meaning, they are trained and informed by the drug companies, or in the U.S. by the FDA and the CDC, all of whose employees are allowed to have stock in, and jobs with drug companies. There are billions of dollars to be made by controlling this disease, which wouldn't be made if there was a cure.

I am very clear that modern, allopathic medicine has some great tools to offer us in the treatment of acute asthma, and many, many lives are saved each and every day because of the treatments made available by it. But curing? The drug companies, despite their publicity to the contrary, stay a long way from that, on purpose.

Pharmaceutical companies sponsor the initial training and continuing education of MD's and DO's, so they end up believing that there is no cure.

Let's have a look at how modern allopathy works for asthma:

❖ In severe, acute cases corticosteroids are used. These prevent the airways from swelling up. These corticosteroids can be in the form of inhaler sprays, through nebulizers, IV's, injection, or in tablet form. Corticosteroids can sometimes save lives. Sometimes they are the wisest choice. However, they tend to be over-used, and they can have very unpleasant side effects, including reduced immune function.

❖ Often leukotriene inhibitor sprays are used on a regular basis to prevent asthmatic episodes. These are usually well tolerated, but they do quadruple the chance of death by asthma.

❖ Bronchiodilators, which can be taken by inhaler, nebulizer, tablets, or by injection, can be very helpful to fend off or reduce an asthma episode. Their effect is short lived.

❖ Allergy shots are used to desensitize individuals to airborne allergens.

❖ Antihistamines are used to prevent the physiological reactions to exposure to allergens.

❖ Oxygen either through a mask or through a nasal cannula provides a temporary, but sometimes valuable degree of relief. However, if used in the long run, this can reduce the rate at which the body makes red blood cells, thus compounding the problem.

Measuring how well you breathe include the following:

❖ Spirometry is the use of a device that measures how much air you can exhale and how forcefully you can breathe out. Spirometry is a good way to see how much your breathing is impaired.

❖ Peak flow meter: This is another way of measuring how forcefully you can breathe out during an attack.

❖ Oximetry: Often referred to as a "Pulse ox". It reads how saturated with oxygen your blood is, which is often expressed as "O_2 sat". The device is be placed on your fingertip to measure the amount of oxygen in your bloodstream.

❖ Your blood may be checked for signs of an infection that might be contributing to an attack. In severe attacks, it may be necessary to sample blood from an artery to determine exactly how much oxygen and _carbon dioxide_ are present in your body.

Chapter 5

Solutions

Strategies to manage Mental and Emotional challenges

First, believe in the possibility that you can be well, regardless of the evidence, regardless of whether you can clearly imagine it now, or not. Regardless of whether you've been working at getting well for days, months, years or decades. It's essential for your mind in helping your body to work well.

Second, in those moments that you are struggling for your life, trust that you'll be okay. Really, just trust. This may or may not be true. But by the same token, to trust that you won't be okay, may or may not be true. But your cells have consciousness and they eavesdrop on your thoughts. Give them instructions you *intend* them to have.

❖ Be calm; allow things to be as they are. Because, you know what? That's the way they are. Resisting how things are, or resisting change just creates resistance. In the body that equals tension. Yes, you may be eager for change, and probably even in a hurry. But start from the here and now. Create your intended life while relaxed, with a free and calm mind.

❖ Be internally still - meditate. Peace creates such great physiology. In other words, when you are peaceful, your body works better. It soothes inflammation, relieves tension, allows detoxification.

❖ Allow your breathing to be as it is. Does that sound nutty? Allow it to be as it is? Clearly you want it to change. But allowing it to be as it is reduces the amount of tension in the body, including the amount of tension in the lungs.

❖ Allow yourself to be with the issues in your life. Don't avoid them. They might or might not go away. You won't forget them by trying to forget them. Be courageous. Imagine you as the biggest, most mature person you can be, standing calmly and confidently in front of any of the issues with which you are faced.

❖ Practice this several times a day. Like everything else in life, it does take practice to be good at it.

Clearing out fungus

If you have fungus in the lungs, whether it is causing asthma or not, it needs to be cleaned out. Find out first. Get diagnosed. If you do, then it's vital to clean it out. Where to start? In the intestines! Because most of the time, most of the fungus in the body is in the intestines. Here's how to get rid of it from there: make sure you're having at least 2-3 bowel movements per day. If you're not, modify your diet, drink more water, and if necessary, take peristalsis-inducing laxatives until you are at 2-3 bowel movements per day. Then start on a charcoal, bentonite, apple pectin combination. This will absorb the crud in the intestines, it will pull out the mucus plugs (mucus tucked into the intestinal folds), biofilm (bacteria or fungal slime), and fecal plaque (left over, dried fecal matter), and you'll poop them out. Depending on your size, take 1-3 tablespoons of the mixture shaken in water. Drink it down quickly and chase it with 1-3 pints of water. Make sure you do this at a time of day when you're not putting nutrients or meds into your mouth, because they will be at least partially absorbed by the mixture. Leave 2 hours after taking the mixture before you eat, or to take any nutrients, foods or meds. Take the mixture at least once a day, and continue for 2 weeks. That will reduce the overall load of fungus in the body, so that antifungals will have an easier time killing the rest of the fungus, and the antifungals will have an easier time reaching whatever fungus may be left in the intestines.

Another valuable helper in this department is colonic irrigation. This will flush out the large intestines. As long as it's done well, it'll be a thorough cleaning of the large intestines. Remember, this won't reach the small intestines.

Next, it's important to take antifungals. The way most physicians treat fungus, is to provide a few days of Fluconazole (a systemic antifungal: this gets all through the body), or Nystatin (a gastro-intestinal antifungal: this should just stay in the GI tract). These prescription antifungals work. The fluconazole is said to be hard on the liver, but I have never seen, nor heard of patients being harmed by it. One problem that I've seen with the use of these, is that they are given without any consideration for what will grow once the fungus is gone. Yes, once again, inside your body is warm and wet. Something IS going to grow! Most often it's fungus, innocuous bacteria, sometimes beneficial bacteria, sometimes harmful bacteria. And the immune system that has not been strong enough to stop fungus from growing, also needs some help.

So my strategy for clearing fungus includes taking antifungals for at least a month while building the immune system and building up a great colony of helpful bacteria (probiotics). But I don't recommend taking the prescription antifungals for a month. For safety's sake, I recommend other antifungals:

- ❖ Colloidal silver 50-100 parts per million, ½ to 2 teaspoonfuls twice a day, depending on your size. Limit use of colloidal silver to one month in any three, it is a mildly toxic metal, and needs time to leave the body.
- ❖ Grapefruit seed extract (NOT grape seed extract, which is also a valuable nutrient, but not an antifungal), 5-20 drops per day, 2-3 times daily.
- ❖ Oil of oregano, tastes awful. It's available in capsules, thankfully. A recent discovery I made was that oil of oregano smeared on the soles of the feet rapidly kills fungus in the blood. I believe any soft areas of skin should work for this. Dose depends upon your size, and capsule size. As far as external application, 4-12 drops 2-3 times daily should do the trick.

There is the possibility that you may feel worse, fatigued, or have flu-like symptoms when killing off fungus. This is because the toxins that the fungus would normally be releasing at a slow rate into your body, are suddenly released all at once when the fungus dies. The best thing to do at this point is to increase your water intake by 50% and take lots of antioxidants for a few days.

Of course once the fungus is killed, it is important to establish a healthy colony of good bacteria in the gut. Most people have heard of acidophilus. Acidophilus is one strain of a family of bacteria called Lactobacillus. That's why you'll sometimes see L. Acidophilus. There are several strains of Lactobacillus that can be taken to improve gastrointestinal function, and there is another major family of bacteria with which we should populate the gut, and that is the Bifidobacter family. Taking a combination of around 30 billion units per 100 pounds of body weight is a good dose. Take this for a month immediately after stopping the antifungals.

You could take the probiotics while you're taking the antifungals as well, I would argue that the antifungals, some of which are also antibiotic, can kill off the good bacteria as well, so it may just be a waste of your money.

Improving your environment

Devices:

Air filtration. This can be integral with heating and air conditioning systems, or they can be stand-alone units. The degree to which filtration works to take particles out of the air depends upon how fine the air filter is and how much air is forced through the filter. Also it is important that as much of the air as possible in the room, house, office, workshop, or warehouse go through the filter. Not the same, small portion of the air being refiltered over and over. So, place a filtration system either by an air conditioning return vent, or in a wide open area, maybe in the middle of your house or workplace.

Ionizers. Ionizers create a negatively charged environment. The more powerful the ionizer, the greater the area effected. Ionizers cause the particles in the air to clump together and these larger clumps of particles can't float in the air, so they fall to the ground, and then we don't breathe them.

Ultraviolet lights. UV light kills bacteria, fungus and viruses. UV lights can be installed in air conditioning systems, they are also available in stand-alone units that use fans to draw air in and past the light.

Ozone generators. Oxygen is stable in the air as O_2. In other words, 2 atoms of oxygen make up the O_2 molecule. Ozone is longer molecules of oxygen, O3 (and sometimes longer chains of oxygen). While ozone does provide protection to the surface of the Earth while it is at high altitudes, it is not safe to breathe it. Ozone breaks down to O_2 very easily, and in doing so it releases energy. It's this release of energy that damages surrounding cells. If ozone is inhaled in high concentrations, and breaks down to O_2 in the lungs, the membranes of the lungs can be damaged. So the use of ozone generators that kill bacteria, fungus, parasites and viruses in a home or work environment should absolutely be restricted to operation when there are no humans, other animals or plants in the room or rooms that are being ozonated.

Some ozone generator sales people have said that it's a nice smell and that it's okay to breathe it in. No, absolutely not! I suggest they are ignorant of the science of the matter.

There are certain air cleaning devices that include some or all the above. I recommend you buy one. How to use it? Get all the plants and animals (including the human animals) out of the house, run the ozone machine overnight. Go back in, holding your breath, switch off the device, then allow half an hour of thorough ventilation before you back in.

Practices:

- ❖ Vacuum your bed. Keep the dust and dust mites out! The fecal matter from dust mites contain their digestive enzymes which are an allergen for many people.
- ❖ Wash sheets, bed covers and pillows. You should know that old pillows weigh sometimes 50% more than when they were new. The additional weight? Skin flakes, dust mites, dust mite fecal matter, and sweat. Lovely!
- ❖ Clean or replace heater and air conditioning vents. These can be prime breeding grounds for mold.
- ❖ Reduce carpet area. Carpets can contain dust, bacteria, fungus, and moisture.
- ❖ Reduce glues, paints, inks, cleaners, bleach, etc. The strong and often toxic fumes can irritate the mucus membranes of the lungs, sometimes causing constriction of bronchioles, and more mucus often gets produced. What's more, the toxins can get into the body, increasing oxidative stress and the overall toxic load.
- ❖ Check for and remove mold from the home, work and school, including in the walls.

❖ Live in a low allergen environment. Make sure to decrease dust, insects (especially cockroaches), dust mites, furry animals, and feathered animals.

For some of us, there may come a time when it becomes worthwhile to move to a different part of the world, where there is less pollen, less mold, less dust, less pollution, and maybe a different climate. It is worth considering.

<u>Dietary Solutions</u>

For asthmatics, it is vital to eliminate foods to which they may be allergic, sensitive or intolerant. Almost any food can be an allergen. Some people are allergic to many foods, while others are allergic to none. But if someone has asthma, it is worth delving into this issue thoroughly, and finding out which foods might be a problem. So far, the laboratory and clinical allergy testing for foods is not as accurate as I would like. So, it is worthwhile excluding certain foods **completely** for a set period of time, and then reintroducing them. If symptoms reduce while the food is excluded, and return when the food is reintroduced, then it is fair to say that there is an allergy, sensitivity or intolerance to it. This method takes time, and is more accurate than any testing. Of course, labs and clinical testers will disagree, but that's their prerogative.

You might ask "Which foods should go first?" or "Which foods should I try avoiding first, to see if it makes a difference?" I'd say cut out all dairy first. You'll be astounded at the difference you feel, in your general well being, in various aspects of your health, and in your symptoms. Here's what I've found about excluding dairy from the diet: whereas reducing by half most foods that cause health problems, reduces the health problems by half, cutting dairy by half, when it causes allergies only reduces the reactions by 10%-30%. If you have an allergic reaction to dairy it needs to be a 100% abstention, for at least a month (the effects of the dairy proteins take a while to be removed from the body) before expecting any significant difference.

Cut out gluten either second or at the same as the dairy. When you exclude gluten from your diet you are more likely to see changes within 2 weeks. Gluten is the most allergenic food. Aside from all the people allergic to gluten, many people simply don't digest it well. Gluten exists in all the grains listed above. Strangely enough when gluten grains are sprouted most people with an intolerance or an allergy can then consume them without a problem. For instance wheat grass juice is generally well tolerated by some celiacs. Experimentation for your self or ones in your care is worthwhile to establish individual susceptibilities.

Make sure that at least most of the food you eat is organically grown. Why? It actually has the nutrients it is supposed to have. AND there are pesticides, herbicides, and growth promoters. The added load of toxicity from these chemicals strains the detoxification system, the immune system and increases inflammation in the body.
Eat as much of your food as possible, raw. I know, you're thinking "Salads?" There are many books describing the

vast number of recipes for raw foods. There are dishes you wouldn't imagine; tasty, varied, and more nutritious. Why? Because in raw food, the nutrients are not destroyed by heat. Raw food diets cure many, many diseases, including diabetes.

A world famous figure in the raw food movement is Victoria Boutenko, whose daughter had asthma until the family switched to a raw food diet. I encourage you to research Victoria's terrific story, and her life-changing work.

Here are a few books that will guide you towards building great health. Not all the recipes are hypoallergenic, but most of them are:

- ❖ Healthful Cuisine, by Anna Maria Clement and Kelly Serbonich
- ❖ Rawesomely Vegan, by Mike Snyder.
- ❖ The Kind Diet, by Alicia Silverstone
- ❖ Vegan Cooking for Carnivores, by Roberto Martin

Yes all of these are books teaching you a plant-based diet. Believe me, that's a vital part of what it takes to get healthy, all the research says that, my patients see that for themselves, you'll find that too. For some of you it may just take some extra desperation to motivate you in that direction. I just hope your resistance to a plant-based diet doesn't kill you.

For those of you who like to eat meat, eventually, when you've recovered yourself, and you'd like to relax your diet, I'd recommend the Paleolithic diet.

Building your immune system

Building your immune function will help your body to dispose of microbes that could irritate your lungs.

Here are a few tips for building your immune system:

❖ Be happy and have a powerful, positive mindset about everything, including your immunity. BELIEVE that you can beat the microbes. FEEL your white blood cells defending you. Visualize yourself in perfect health. You think it's mumbo jumbo? Try it. Practice it. You'll notice a difference, I did, and many of my patients have. Your cells have consciousness, they eavesdrop on your thoughts. Teach them well.

❖ Exercise (but not excessive amounts of extensive exercise. Make it short, and vigorous).

❖ Eat fresh, live, organically grown food.

❖ Get fresh air and sunshine.

❖ Wash your hands.

❖ Avoid smoking, drinking alcohol, and other drugs.

❖ Avoid vaccines (Yes, because of the toxicity and immune load the vaccines present, they leave people MORE susceptible to disease, including infectious diseases and asthma).

❖ Use combinations of the following to help build your immune system:

  o Vit. C

- Vit. A/β-Carotene
- Echinacea
- Ginseng (but not if you have a red tongue, this indicates heat, and ginseng is very heating.)
- Siberian Ginseng (a completely different plant from Korean, Chinese, American, Panax Ginseng)
- Goldenseal
- Wolfberry/Lycium/Goji
- Astragalus
- Cat's Claw/Uňa de Gato
- Probiotics
- Spirulina
- Aloe Vera

Solutions to the vaccine issue

Healing from the damage of vaccines can take a whole lot of work, and much of the content of the second half of this book, the detoxification, the hypoallergenic diet, removing the toxic metals, can all be used towards it.

Given that some people die from vaccines, and some are severely handicapped following vaccination, it is clear that not all vaccine damage is recoverable. But most is. The vast extend of damage, and therefore the vast extent of work needed to repair vaccine damage can't be covered in the context of this book, or our asthma recovery workshops, and really deserves its own context, in other words, books, conferences and treatment programs, etc. dedicated to resolving all the problems caused by vaccines.

Just be assured there are legal professionals around the country who are ready and willing to work with you on the exemptions that are already available, so that you can go to work, including in the military, including in hospitals, and your children can go to school, without having vaccines.

Detoxifying toxic metals

The most common toxic metals to cause problems that increase bacterial and fungal infections in the body are mercury, and aluminium. To rid the body of these, start by avoiding exposure.

Mercury and aluminum have a high affinity for neurological tissue, in other words, they like to bond with the brain and the nerves, so it is important that the substances you take to pull them out of storage and into circulation, create a stronger bond with the metals than the metals do with the brain (and other tissues). (Just like if you glue a wooden block to wallpaper. You pull the block, and the wallpaper comes off the wall because the glue is stronger than the wallpaper paste.) Then having pulled the toxic metals into circulation, they can be passed out of the body in the urine and the stool.

Taking toxic metals out of storage in the tissues, into circulation can cause problems by allowing the metals to contact other tissues. This can be controlled, so I recommend that chelation and detoxification of toxic metals, should be done with the help of a health care provided experienced in the process.

Here are a few chelating and detoxification agents:

Cilantro	for mercury
Glutathione	for mercury
Selenium	for mercury
Zinc	for cadmium
DMPS	for aluminum and mercury
DMSA	for mercury
EDTA	for aluminum, lead and mercury

Please seek the help of physicians who deal with detoxification of toxic metals to deal with this kind of toxicity, as certain chelation agents are safer than others, and chelating slowly is much safer than doing it quickly.

<u>Reducing phlegm</u>

There are certain foods which are worth avoiding, if you intend to reduce the phlegm in your lungs. These include:

1. Dairy (I don't mean eggs)
2. Sugar
3. Oranges/orange juice
4. Gluten (for some people, this increases phlegm)

Avoid being in damp and moldy environments. Make sure that where you live and work has dry carpet, dry walls, dry ceiling and dry furniture, and a good roof. Keep it all in good repair. Use a dehumidifier. Use an air purifier like the ones mentioned above.

Chinese herbal medicine has many formulae to clear phlegm. Find a Doctor of Oriental Medicine/Acupuncture Physician to get a prescription. They will get one suitable for your overall condition, including for the phlegm issue.

Acupuncture is also a very good choice for activating the body to clear phlegm.

Breathing techniques

There are two anatomical mechanisms that pull air into the lungs.

One is the diaphragm. The diaphragm is a dome shaped muscle below the thoracic organs: the heart and lungs, and above the abdominal organs: the liver, kidneys, bladder, stomach, intestines, spleen, and reproductive organs. When the diaphragm contracts, it flattens out, so it pushes down on the abdominal organs and the belly moves outward. At the same time it pulls down on the thoracic organs, enlarging the space above the diaphragm, which means that air rushes into this extra space through the nose or mouth, down through the trachea, and into the lungs.

The other mechanism is the movement of the ribs. The muscles between the ribs, called the intercostals muscles, pull the ribs closer together, and because of their shape they lift up a little. When the ribs lift up, the space within the chest enlarges, and air rushes in through the nose or mouth, down through the trachea, and into the lungs to fill that extra space.

Most people only use their ribs to breathe and not their diaphragm. That means that they don't get as much air as they might.

Notice if when you breathe, whether your chest rises and falls, or whether your belly goes in and out. Or both. None of these styles of breathing are wrong or right, but if you are like most people, your chest will fall and rise.

To increase the amount of air that you take in, make sure that that your belly expands as air goes in, and contracts as air goes out. To create a more complete breath, start by breathing in so that your belly expands. Once your belly is fully expanded, keep it expanded, and breathe in using your ribs, so that they rise. Then breathing out, allow your ribs to fall, and then allow your belly to contract.

I cannot emphasize enough how important exercise is for expanding your breathing capacity. Not only do you strengthen your breathing muscles, but you make your skeletal muscles more efficient so that under normal circumstances they aren't using as much oxygen, you build up reserves of myoglobin (a substance in the muscles that stores oxygen ready for use in exercise), and you build up your number of red blood cells so that the oxygen carrying capacity of the blood is increased. Both intense, short periods of exercise, and endurance exercise, are important. Start gently, under professional supervision. Gradually and very gradually, build up. Find something that is fun for you, so that you stick to it.

There are some extra breathing techniques that you can do to help your breathing. Try this:

1. Choose a place and time where you can relax. Breathe most of the way out, and hold that position; for a while, don't breathe. Don't strain.
2. When you feel a stronger urge to breathe in, breathe in.

This exercise increases your body's ability to breathe. You can repeat this several times a day. Try this during an attack. See if it eases things up. The temporary buildup of CO_2 should ease your breathing there and then.

When you are having an attack, don't try to over-breathe. Don't try to pant.

1. Breathe slowly, taking larger than average breaths.
2. Breathe in, and without blocking your throat,
3. Hold your breath for 5-10 seconds,
4. Breathe out, and once again without blocking your throat,
5. Hold for 5-10 seconds. You may find this a very helpful technique. I remember that it helped me.

Other stuff that helps

Acupuncture

There are many different styles of acupuncture, different levels of skill of the doctor, and every patient has their own level of susceptibility to the treatment.

For most people acupuncture is a powerful tool for building health, including lung health. One tip, though: don't expect your acupuncturist necessarily to treat you on the "Lung Meridian" (that's the line of acupuncture points that go to and through the lungs). For instance, when I had treatment that worked very well for my breathing, my acupuncturist treated my Heart meridian. That in turn, benefited my lungs.

Have at least one treatment per week at the beginning, reducing in frequency as you improve. Carry on with treatment for at least a year. If after 10 treatments you should be seeing at least a little improvement. If not, switch to another acupuncturist and start the year of treatment again. It really can make that much of a difference to change to a new doctor. There are so many acupuncture points, literally billions of different point combination permutations, so there are many different treatment protocols for any given disease.

Chinese herbal medicine

There are many different Chinese herbal remedies, and several that address lung health. In Oriental medicine we have strange sounding diagnoses, for instance: Yin deficiency, Yang deficiency, phlegm, damp-heat, wind heat, wind cold. These and many more describe the behavior of the organs, and the interaction between the organs and pathogenic factors. Not everyone with asthma will have the same Oriental diagnosis. A skilled doctor of Oriental medicine, just like a skilled acupuncture doctor, or a skilled homeopath will discern the difference between one type of asthma and another, and apply that information in the prescribing of the treatment.

A study done in China in the 1990's showed that many asthmatics are producing more adrenaline than they are using with muscular movement, for instance, when watching TV, or paying video games. This produces heat in the body. Their solution? Reduce T.V.,

Another Oriental medical study showed that cold showers worked well to clear asthma!

Homeopathy

Homeopathy is the use of natural substances that have been extremely diluted. It is very safe, easy to administer, but a real challenge to prescribe correctly. Find a good homeopath and have them work on you for at least a year. It can take a while to nail down and fine tune the right remedy. But when it works well, it can be miraculous.

Chiropractic/osteopathy

It is vital that the bones, discs and soft tissue of the spine are all healthy, have good tone and are well aligned in order for optimum nerve supply to the organs. This includes the lungs. Sometimes soft tissue and bone manipulation of the neck and upper thoracic area can substantially help breathing.

I had an accident in martial arts training which damaged my neck. Immediately my breathing was impaired. My friend Dr. Samuels, a skilled osteopath, worked on my neck and I got immediate and permanent relief.

At least be checked for your spinal health. Once again, there are some chiropractors and osteopaths that are better suited to your own body's needs than others. They all work differently; they have different style. Ask friends, shop around, find one you like, one whose treatment benefits seem to last.

Echinacea

Echinacea, when taken as a liquid, acts as a bronchiodilator. It also is beneficial to the immune system. When you take it, it should produce a strong fizz/tingle in your mouth.

Lobelia

Lobelia can be helpful in lung health, but I'd recommend use only under the supervision of a herbalist.

Magnesium

Magnesium relaxes smooth muscle tissue. Smooth muscle tissue exists in the lining of the intestines, in the iris of the eye, in the skin, and surrounding the blood vessels (that's one reason magnesium reduces blood pressure).

Smooth muscle tissue also exists around the tubes to the lungs, so there they can restrict or increase the amount of air that is allowed into and out off the lungs. Taking magnesium will relax these muscles so that the airways open and allow more air in and out. If you're wanting this effect, it's important to not take calcium with the magnesium, because calcium tightens smooth muscle tissue. Increase the amount of magnesium from 200mg/day/100lb of body weight by 50mg-100mg each day, until you get a little bit of diarrhea, then reduce the dose by about 100mg. This is a dosage strategy called "...to bowel tolerance". In this case it's "Magnesium to bowel tolerance". If your blood pressure drops so that either number is less than 90 on the top, or 50 on the bottom, you then need to reduce the amount of magnesium you're taking.

Chapter 6
Finally

I have given you a lot of tools with which to improve your and your family's health. It may seem simple to you, it may seem overwhelming. If it seems overwhelming, just make gradual changes. Don't only do one thing at a time, drop it and start something else. That's a recipe for failure. Start with one of my suggestions, then when you've got that down, add another, then three, etc.

You know, drug companies aren't going to come to your rescue. There may be temporary, and much needed relief, but remember, a drug isn't going to cure you. As far as the drug companies are concerned, there is no money in a cure.

Health can take a great deal of work. It involves changing and fine-tuning every area of your life, physical and mental. And persist; it took me years, and it was so worth it. I just wished I'd started years before. You will too. So start today. Good luck.

If you need extra help with restoring lung health, join us on one of our lung health retreats. It's will be the experience of a lifetime. Personal consultations are available too. Contact us at:

contact@NaturalFamilyPhysicians.com

or call us at

239-540-1220.

Be well!

www.ingramcontent.com/pod-product-compliance
Lightning Source LLC
Chambersburg PA
CBHW071304170526
45165CB00003B/1409